BODY TALK

MIND AND MATTER

THE BRAIN AND NERVOUS SYSTEM

JENNY BRYAN

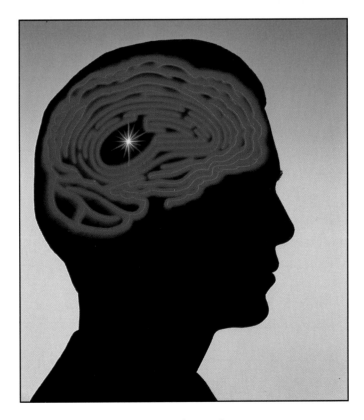

Wayland

B O D Y T A L K

BREATHING

REPRODUCTION

DIGESTION

MIND AND MATTER

MOVEMENT

SOUND AND VISION

SMELL, TASTE AND TOUCH

THE PULSE OF LIFE

Editor: Catherine Baxter
Series Design: Loraine Hayes
Consultant: Dr Tony Smith – Associate Editor of the *British Medical Journal*
Cover and title page: Special effects photograph of the human brain.

First published in 1993 by Wayland (Publishers) Ltd.
61 Western Road
Hove, East Sussex, BN3 1JD, England.
© Copyright 1992 Wayland Publishers Ltd.

British Library Cataloguing in Publication Data
Bryan, Jenny
Mind and Matter: Brain and Nervous System. –
(Body Talk Series)
I. Title II. Series
612.8

ISBN 07502 0491 5

Typeset by Key Origination, 1 Commercial Road, Eastbourne
Printed in Italy by G. Canale & C.S.p.A., Turin
Bound in France by A.G.M.

CONTENTS

INTRODUCTION

The brain is an organ like the heart and lungs – but the mind isn't. You can't see or touch the mind. Yet, it makes us who we are. It is our mental ability that puts human beings at the top of the evolutionary ladder. Physically, we are much weaker than many other animals. But our ability to think and reason allows us to outwit other species that could tear us to pieces in a face-to-face fight.

As individuals, our minds also decide what sort of people we are. The things we like to do, how we behave towards other people, whether we laugh a lot, or cry, whether we are good at understanding and remembering things, whether we are cruel or kind, are decided by our minds.

Of course, the way we are brought up also affects who and what we are. We learn about right and wrong from what we see and hear. A child may be born with a happy personality. But if all it sees and experiences is cruelty, it may become sad and be cruel to other people.

Although the mind is not an organ, the cells which control the way we think are in the brain. We know less about how the brain works than any other part of the body. In fact, some parts are a complete mystery. But we are starting to understand which parts of the brain control different activities and how they work together.

This is also helping us to understand what makes us so different from other animals. For example, the parts of the brain which control breathing, heartbeat and reflex movement are very similar. But the parts of the brain which deal with thinking and reasoning are more developed in humans than in animals.

Fish have a much better sense of smell than us because they need it to find food. Similarly, amphibians and birds have wonderful eyesight to help them track down prey. It's lucky for us that we are better thinkers, or life in the animal kingdom would be a lot harder!

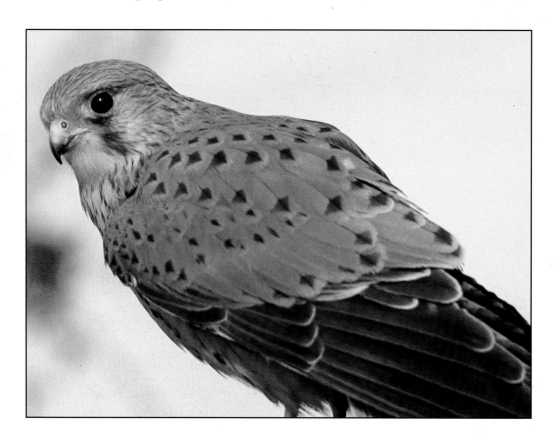

Kestrels and other birds of prey have better eyesight than humans because, when flying high above the ground, they need to spot mice and other tasty snacks. However, humans are better thinkers.

OPPOSITE How we are treated when we are young affects the kind of people we grow into.

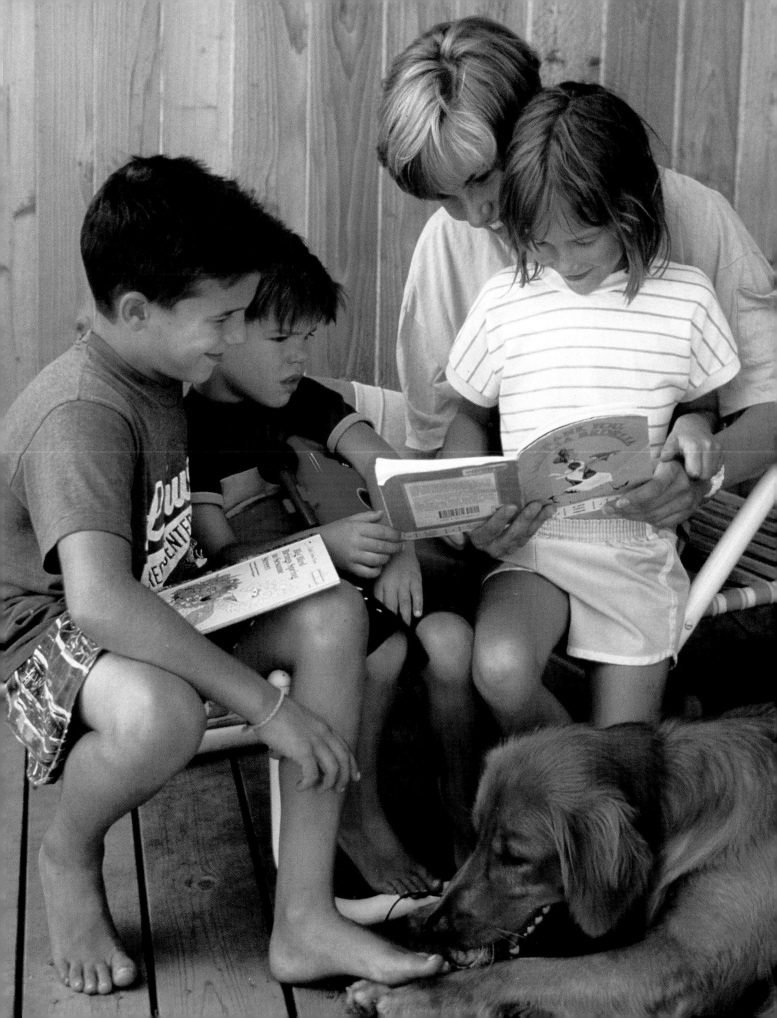

THE BRAIN

An adult brain weighs about 1.4 kilograms. It is soft and squidgy and, without the bony skull which covers it, the brain would be easily damaged. It sits on a stalk called the brain stem. Further down, this becomes the spinal cord which runs right down the back of the body. Together, the brain and the spinal cord make up the central nervous system.

The surface of the human brain is ridged so it looks rather like a huge walnut. Rat and mouse brains are smooth. Cleverer animals such as cats, dogs, and monkeys have small ridges. But ours are by far the biggest! The ridges allow more brain cells to be packed into the head than if the surface was smooth and flat.

If you cut the brain down the middle, back to front – you would be left with two halves that looked the same. The halves are joined together by a wide band of nerve fibres so that one side knows what the other is doing.

THE HUMAN BRAIN

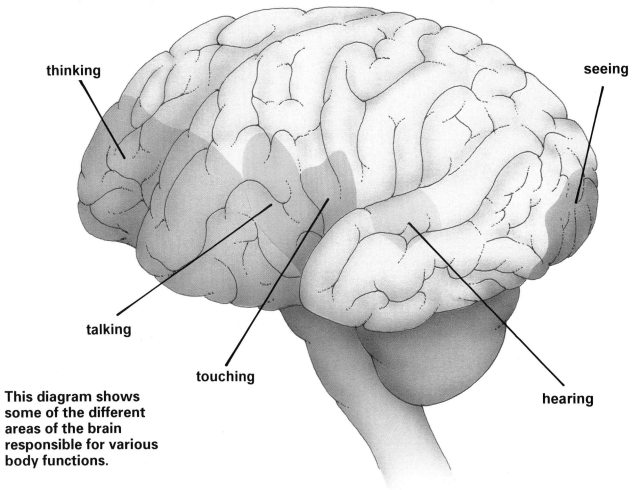

thinking

seeing

talking

touching

hearing

This diagram shows some of the different areas of the brain responsible for various body functions.

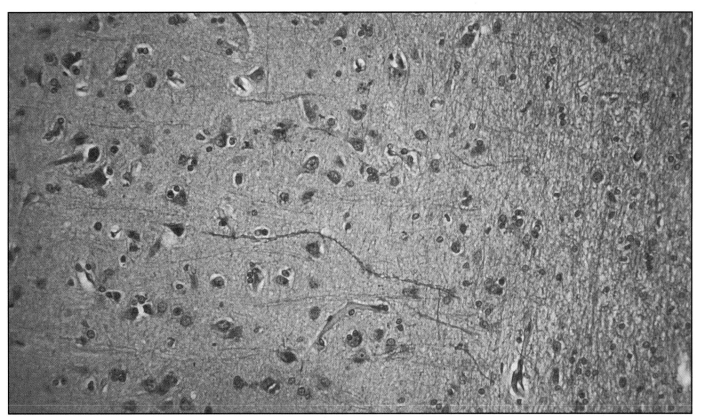

A section of the human cerebral cortex containing grey matter (right) and white matter (left). False mauve colouring has been added so that you can tell them apart.

The outer layer of the human brain is called the cerebral cortex. It is just a few millimetres thick. This is where many of the brain cells are and it is where we do most of our thinking. Because the cells are pinkish grey, the cerebral cortex is known as the grey matter. The cells in the left side look after language and speech and they tell the right side when to move. The cells on the right side control movement in the left side of the body.

Below the cerebral cortex is the white matter. It contains millions of long nerve fibres which carry messages between cells in different parts of the brain. It looks white because the fibres have a white coating, called myelin.

Over millions of years, the human brain has developed so that one part deals with information from the eyes, another with information from the ears and so on. There is some overlap. But scientists have discovered, for example, that information about seeing is dealt with in the cerebral cortex at the back of the brain, hearing at the sides and speech nearer to the front.

Running down the middle of the brain, deep into the core, is the limbic system which is in charge of our emotions.

The brain stem controls activities which we don't have to think about in order for them to happen – heart-rate, blood-pressure, breathing, swallowing and sneezing. At the back of this is a bulge called the cerebellum. This processes information from muscles and from the balance system in the ear, enabling us to move smoothly and quickly without even thinking about it.

BRAIN MYSTERIES

Some parts of the brain, especially in the core, are a complete mystery to us. We just don't know what they do. Nor do we know how different parts of the brain work together to give each of us our own personality. Scientists are still doing experiments to try and find this out.

FIRST THOUGHTS

The brain and spinal cord are the first major parts of the body to form after a sperm and an egg meet (conception). Long before an embryo looks like a human being, a central core of tissue can be seen which will be the spinal cord. The bulge at one end of this will be the brain.

Before a baby is even born, millions of links are formed between the nerves in the brain and spinal cord. It's a bit like building a complete road system. You need motorways, dual carriageways, smaller roads, lanes and paths for the system to be really effective.

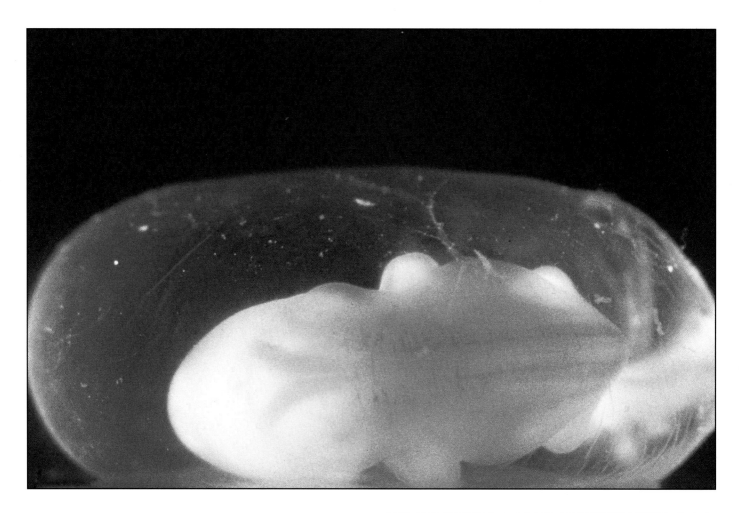

At just eight weeks, the brain and spinal cord can be clearly seen in this human foetus, viewed from the back with the head to the left, and the limb buds centre and right.

EARLIEST MEMORIES

What are your earliest memories? Most people can remember things that happened when they were about two or three years old. A special outing to the countryside may stick in their mind (OPPOSITE). Or they may remember some daily activity, such as playing in the park or walking to school, because they did it so often.

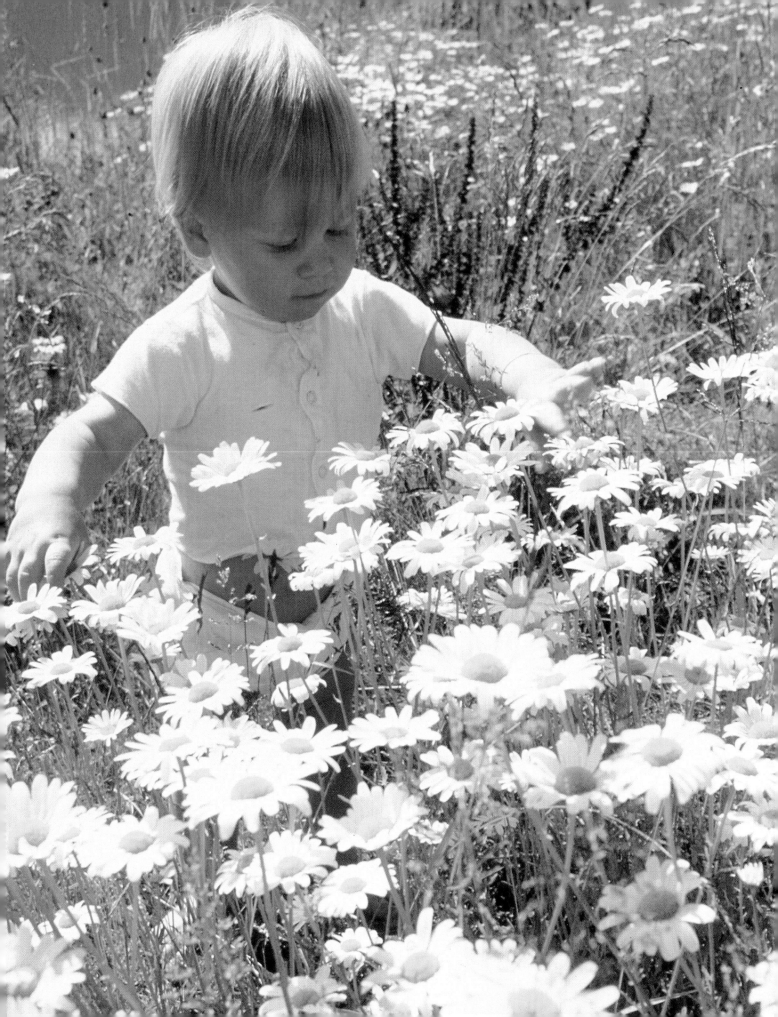

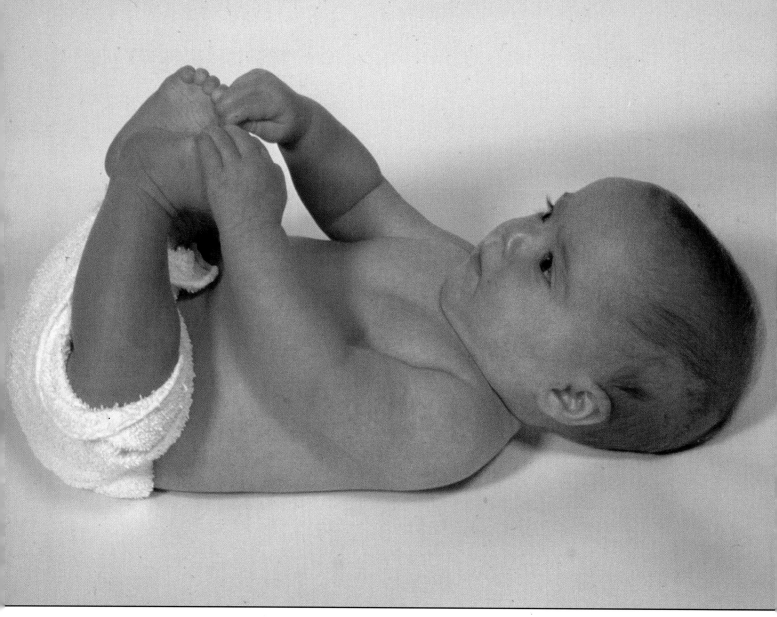

At five months, this baby is just starting to explore his surroundings – beginning with his feet!

Brain cells are made deep in the brain and move outwards to other parts. They go along pathways made of cells called glial cells. These pathways act as a sort of scaffolding. When they get to the cerebral cortex they send out fibres to connect with other parts of the brain. These also use the glial cell scaffolding to get round. The scaffolding is later destroyed.

Just as roads need repair and maintenance so do nerve pathways. They can die if they aren't used or if they are damaged. Luckily, the body makes far more brain cells than it needs. So it doesn't matter if some die. But, if too many die, the body can't work properly.

No one knows exactly when babies start to think. Even in the womb they are probably aware of their surroundings. But who knows what babies think about when they come kicking and screaming into the world? For the first few months they just eat and sleep. Only when their eyes start to focus and they discover their hands and feet, can babies begin to make decisions to move about and explore the world around them.

Throughout this time, nerve pathways are growing and being broken down to keep pace with the baby's needs. For example, different pathways are needed for crawling and walking and for gurgling and talking.

NERVES

There are about 10 billion nerve cells in a human brain. They are called neurones. There are many types of neurone. Sensory neurones carry information from all over the body into the spinal cord and the brain. Motor neurones carry messages back from the brain to the arms, legs, heart, lungs and other organs. Other neurones act as the 'go-betweens' from sensory to motor nerves.

Each neurone has a cell body which contains all the things you usually find in a cell, including the nucleus in overall charge, and the mitochondria which make energy.

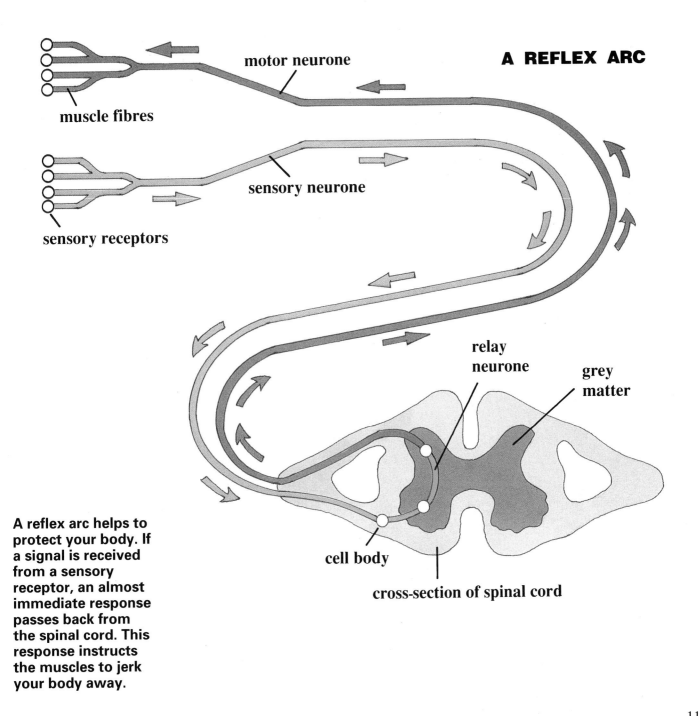

A REFLEX ARC

motor neurone

muscle fibres

sensory neurone

sensory receptors

relay neurone

grey matter

cell body

cross-section of spinal cord

A reflex arc helps to protect your body. If a signal is received from a sensory receptor, an almost immediate response passes back from the spinal cord. This response instructs the muscles to jerk your body away.

Coming out of the cell body are the long fibres which carry messages to and from the brain and spinal cord. The pieces of fibre that carry messages to the cell body are called dendrites. The pieces that carry them away from the cell body are called axons.

Messages are carried down nerve fibres as electrical signals. The end of each fibre splits into lots of nerve endings. When a signal reaches a nerve ending it cannot just jump to the next nerve. It needs to be carried across the gap, called the synapse, by chemicals. These chemicals are called neurotransmitters and there are several different types.

One neuron can be connected to as many as 10, 000 others, so there are literally millions of synapses in the nervous system all needing chemical neurotransmitters.

However, the links between different nerves are not fixed. They change according to how much they are used. Like a country path, if they are used a lot they make a permanent track. But if they aren't used, they become over-grown and impossible to get through.

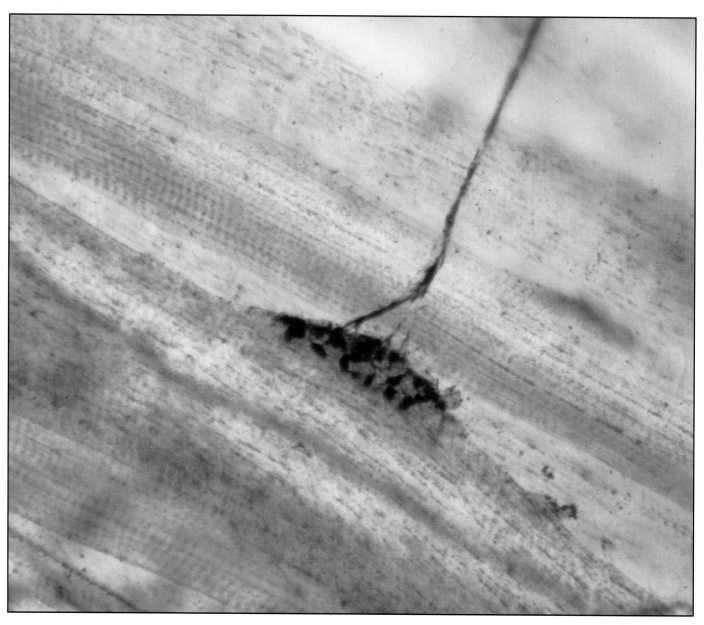

A nerve fibre enters a muscle. It is carrying all the information the muscle needs to make it move.

WHEN THE MESSAGES CAN'T GET THROUGH

If the brain can't make enough of one of the vital neurotransmitters, the messages which it sends to other parts of the body can become jumbled. People with Parkinson's disease – such as the boxer, Muhammed Ali (right) – don't make enough of a neurotransmitter called dopamine. This means that the messages to their arms and legs are garbled and they cannot control their movements. They shake and their speech may become rather slurred.

People with Parkinson's disease can take drugs to replace the missing dopamine. But the drugs don't work as well as the real chemical.

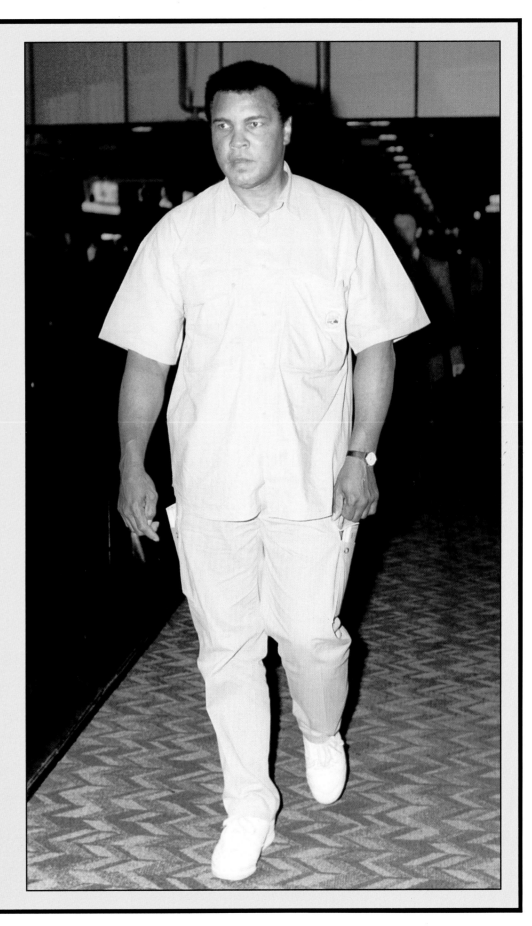

MEMORY

If you bang your head really hard, you usually can't remember what happened to you. You forget all the things just before and during the accident. Memories of things that have just happened are wiped out but older memories stay.

We seem to have two kinds of memory. Short-term memories are things that happened today. Long-term memories are things that happened yesterday, last month, last year and as long ago as we can remember.

The brain processes information about things that happen all the time. Some things are stored in the long-term memory banks while other things are soon forgotten.

As we get older, the storage system may go wrong. Some elderly people cannot remember recent events. But they can still remember things that happened when they were children. Something stops short-term memories from being stored in the long-term banks.

You may need to be very patient with your elderly relatives and tell them things over and over again. It's not their fault that their memories aren't as good as they used to be.

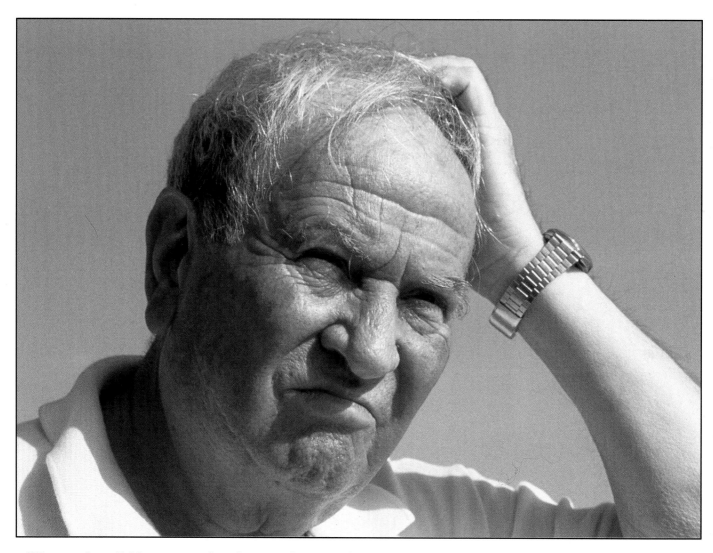

"Now, what did I come to the shops to buy . . . .?"

It's even worse for people who lose all their memory. They cannot lead normal lives. They see a piece of paper and a pen. But they do not know what they are for. Even if someone tells them, they won't remember. So they will never be able to write. They have no old memories and they cannot make any new ones.

There is no single memory centre in the brain. But if parts of the limbic system are damaged, people lose their memories. So it must be important in memory processing.

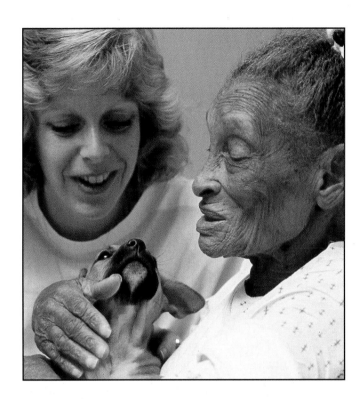

Odd things such as family photographs, old diaries and even much loved pets can help jog an elderly person's memory.

IMPROVING YOUR MEMORY

You can learn all sorts of tricks to help you remember things. For example, if you are revising for an exam you can learn key words that will remind you of large chunks of information. If you want to remember this chapter, the key words to memorize are 'short-term' and 'long-term'!

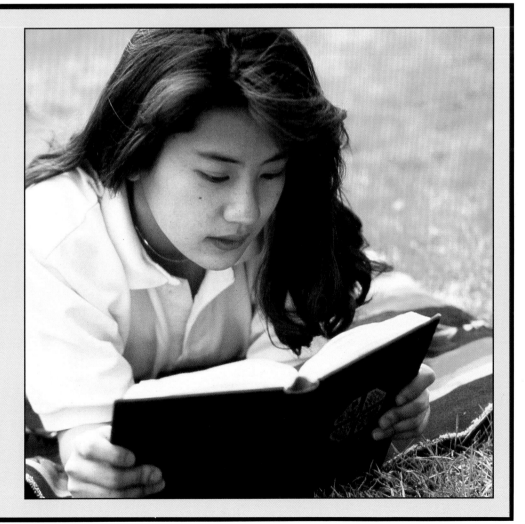

WHO AM I?

No two people are quite the same. Even identical twins have different personalities. But, like it or not, most of us are a bit like our parents! We cannot avoid it.

Your physical and mental make-up are largely decided before you are born. The cells in your brain contain the same genes as the cells in the rest of your body and you inherit half of them from your father and half from your mother. It is your genes which hold the blueprint for everything that goes on in your body.

Just as you rarely look exactly like one or other of your parents, so you will not have exactly the same personality. You may inherit certain skills, such as the ability to draw, to be good at sports or to be musical. But unless you are shown how to use the skills you won't know they are there.

This is why learning is so important. You start to learn when you are only a few weeks old. A baby first learns to recognize its parents. It soon discovers that if it cries someone will come to see what is wrong.

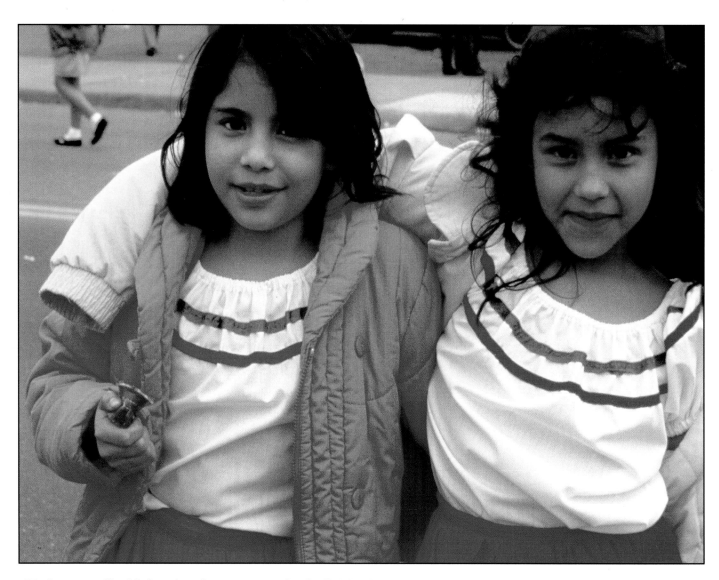

Twins may find it harder than most to be individuals, especially if they dress alike.

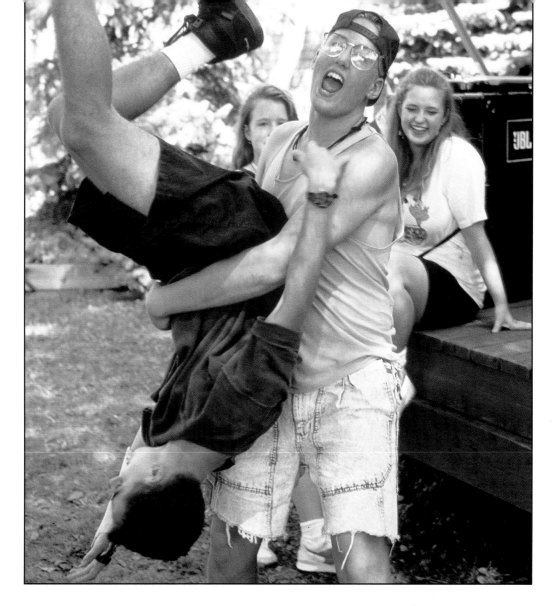

People who are very outgoing and talkative are called extroverts. Quieter, shyer people are called introverts. Which category do you think these people belong to?

You learn some things without even realizing it. You see things going on around you and remember them. You aren't born with attitudes and opinions. These are shaped by the people around you – your family and friends. You have to be taught right from wrong. People have different ideas about what behaviour is acceptable. For example, if a child is brought up in a country at war, he or she may think that it is normal to carry a gun and, if they have seen adults do it, to shoot someone if they disagree with them. Compare that with a child brought up in a loving family. He or she is more likely to feel safe and confident and have no need to be violent.

Some people are more outgoing than others. They talk a lot and they like to be with other people as much as possible. They are called extroverts.

Other people are quieter and shyer. They may be just as happy but they probably prefer to spend considerably more time on their own. They are sometimes called introverts.

It isn't better to be extrovert or introvert. What is important is that you are happy with your life.

AUTISM

Some children cannot talk and play with others. They stay on their own and don't mix. They don't even respond to their families. It's as if there is an invisible wall around them. They are autistic.

If autistic children do not have treatment they will never lead normal lives. But if they are not too badly affected they can be shown how to mix with other people.

INTELLIGENCE

Who is the most intelligent person you can think of? Einstein? Beethoven? Picasso? Marie Curie? All of these people did remarkable things. But how can you compare the mind of a scientist with that of a musician or a painter? Their skills are so very different.

We measure intelligence using tests that check our language skills, ability to count and spatial awareness (how we see things in relation to one another). They are called intelligence quotient (IQ) tests. But experts disagree over the value of such tests. Your intelligence isn't supposed to change – it's something you are born with, something you inherit. But if you do a lot of tests you can learn how to get better scores. So how can IQ tests be reliable?

Today's children score an average 105 in IQ tests, compared with 100 scored by their grandparents. Does this mean they are more intelligent or that they are just better at doing IQ tests? A child of seven or eight can use a computer but many adults can't. Are the children more intelligent? Or is it the way they have been taught.

Children can be intelligent but if they do not have a good education they will not do as well as they could have done. They are less likely to get good jobs.

Before they go to school, girls have higher IQs than boys. But that's because they have better language skills; they understand and can use more words. In fact, right up to puberty, girls learn more quickly than boys.

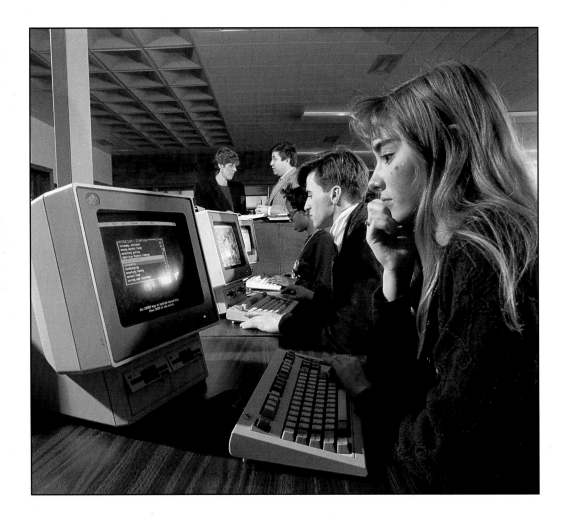

LEFT Being able to use a computer doesn't mean you are cleverer than someone who can't. But in our high-tech world it certainly helps!

RIGHT This robot is hard at work in a nuclear power station in the USA. It can do the work of ten people and it won't be harmed by radiation if there is a leak. Do you think the robot is intelligent? What about the people who designed it?

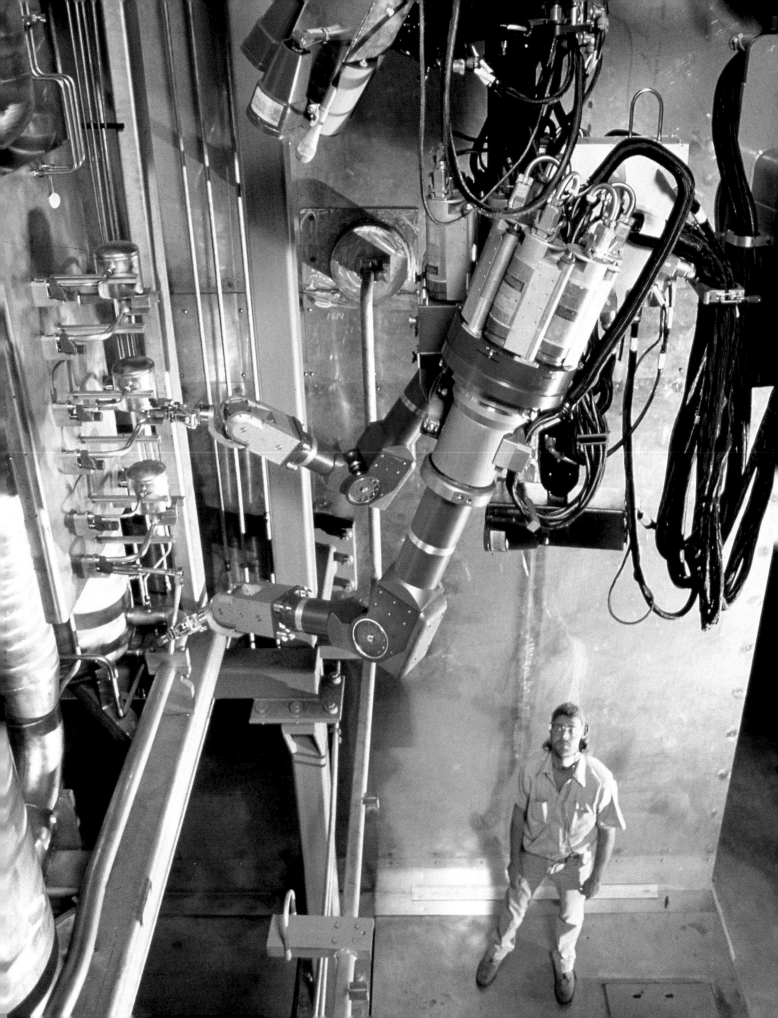

So as you can see, intelligence is very difficult to measure. Being clever or being good at something like art or music is no guarantee of success in life. People have to learn how to use their skills in a way that makes them needed by society. And they have to know how to fit in with society's changing demands.

Forty years ago factories and offices had dozens of people doing jobs which today can be done in half the time by machines such as computers. Skills that guaranteed someone a job in the 1960s may be quite different from those needed to get a job in the 1990s.

PRODIGIES

A prodigy is a child who has developed a special skill at a very early age. For example, a child of five or six who can play the violin at concerts, or a child of twelve who can pass very difficult maths exams. It is easy to imagine that it must be wonderful being a prodigy. However, very gifted children often have problems mixing with children of their own age. Usually this is because they simply aren't interested in the same kinds of things. You could say they are too clever for their own good.

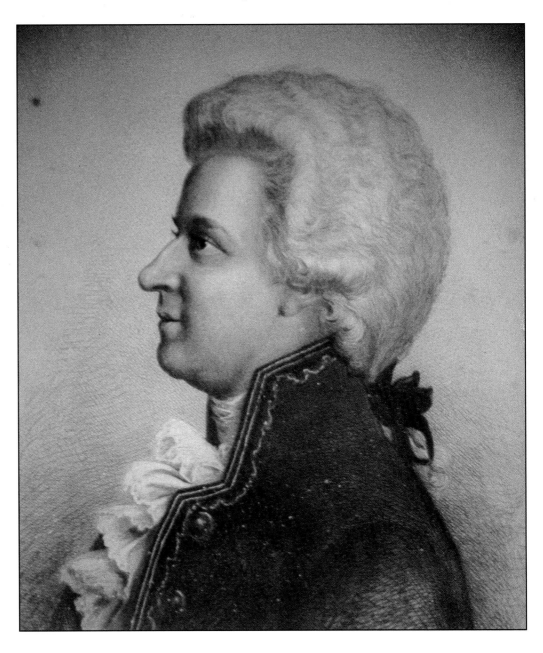

There have been many child prodigies in music, but none more famous than Wolfgang Amadeus Mozart. He could play the harpsichord at the age of three, and was composing music by the time he was five.

FINDING OUT ABOUT PEOPLE

Do you stare at people in wheelchairs? Or do you walk around people who seem to be a bit 'odd'? Most of us find people with disabilities embarrassing. We aren't sure how to cope with them. We might make a fool of ourselves if we try to help them. So what do we do? We do nothing.

Some people are born with physical or mental disabilities. Others become disabled because of an accident or a disease. In many cases it is brain damage that is the cause of the problem. Nerve cells in the brain have been destroyed or nerve pathways have been blocked or broken. Sometimes the damage affects people physically, so they cannot move properly or their eyesight or hearing is bad. Other people are affected mentally so they cannot think properly. The most unfortunate people have brain damage that leaves them mentally and physically disabled.

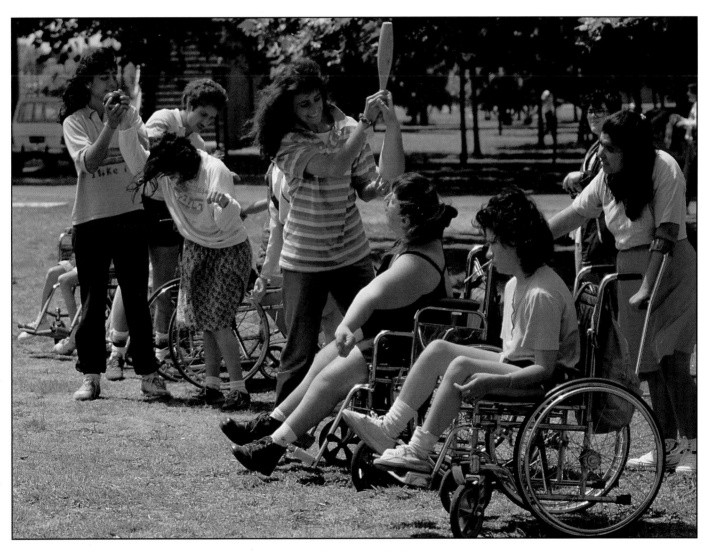

Many disabled people take part in sports and other activities just like anyone else.

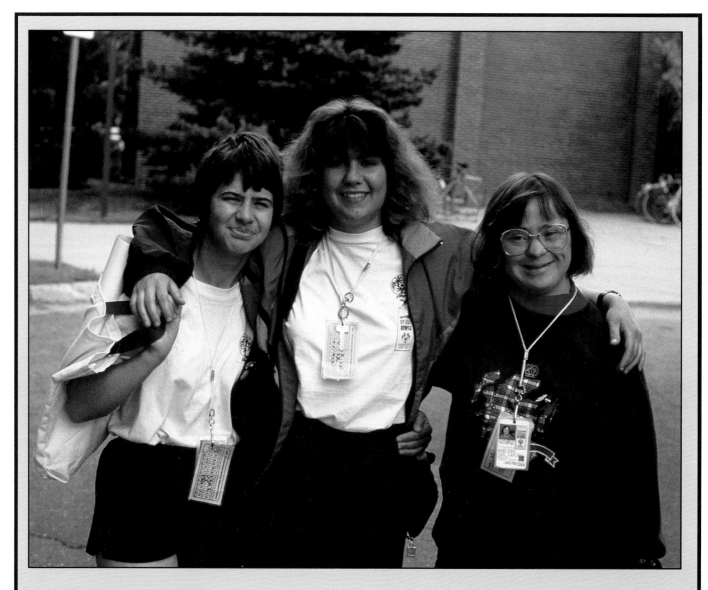

DOWN'S SYNDROME

Some children are born with physical and mental problems because something went wrong with their cells when they were in the womb. They may have too many of the chromosomes which carry genes. This is what happens in Down's syndrome. People with Down's syndrome have rather flat faces and their eyes are slanted. They often have heart problems. They tend to have very happy personalities but they usually need extra help with their school work and some aspects of daily life.

Never assume that because someone is in a wheelchair that they are stupid. They are as clever or bright as you. Being deaf or blind doesn't stop people from passing exams, climbing mountains, even running marathons. Someone who has mental problems can still learn how to look after themselves and to take part in sports and games and other lessons. They may need more help, but they can get just as much fun out of life as the rest of us. They can be just as hurt or unhappy too, especially if people are cruel or unkind to them because of their disabilities.

People do not become disabled because they have done something wrong. But they do need help – not ignorance or pity – to get the most out of their lives.

MIND OVER MATTER

Have you ever seen anyone walk over hot coals or lie on a bed of nails without it hurting? Some people seem to be able to train their minds to block out pain even when they are doing something which would hurt the rest of us very much.

In the mid 1960s, scientists tried to work out how we feel pain. They discovered the 'gate theory' which helps to explain why some people can put up with more pain than others.

Suppose you drop a heavy book on your toe. Messages are immediately sent up the nerves in your leg into your spinal cord, ready to go to your brain. But first they must go through a 'gate'. At this gate in the spinal cord the messages from your toe must compete with messages coming from other parts of the body. There will also be information coming down the spinal cord from the brain which may open the gate wider or close it.

If, when you hurt your toe, you rub it quickly this will send soothing messages up to the gate so it begins to close. Suppose also that when you hurt your toe your friends are watching. You don't want them to think you're making a fuss so your brain will probably send messages down to the gate to override the pain messages on their way up. Thus the final message that gets through the gate and is sent to the brain may be quite different from that which left your toe.

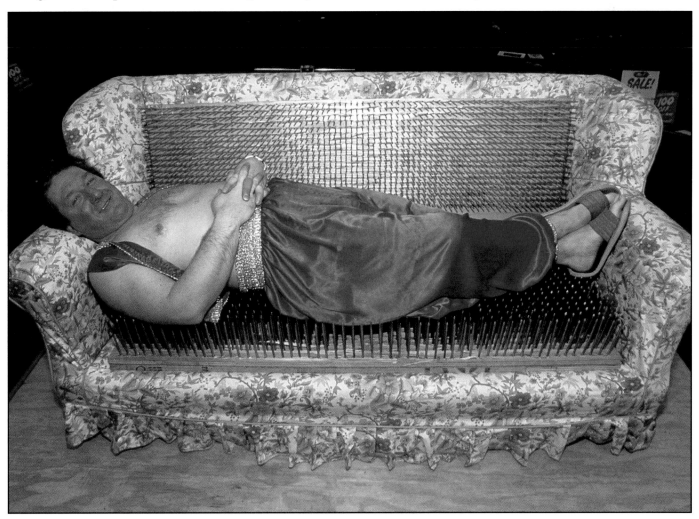

This stuntman is lying on a bed of nails. He has trained his mind to block out pain.

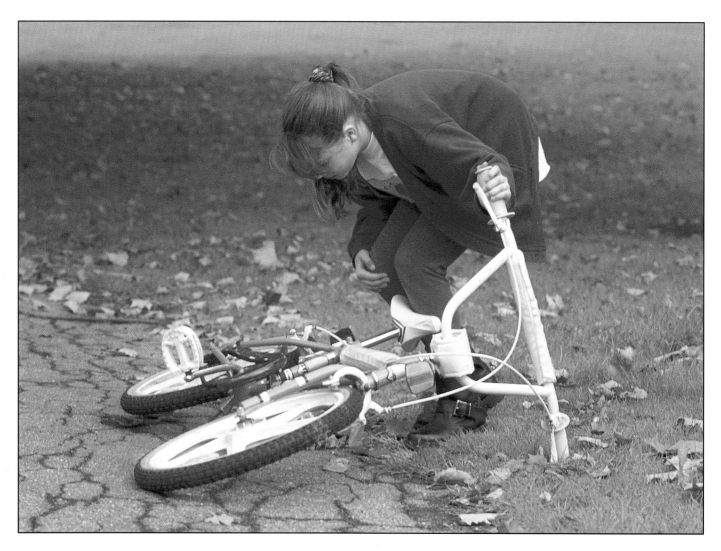

By rubbing her knee, this girl is reducing the pain messages going to her brain.

SEEING YOURSELF BETTER

The pain gate helps to explain why some people can put up with quite severe pain simply by willing it not to hurt. It also helps to explain why some people cannot.

For example some people suffer long periods of back pain, but their X-rays show there is very little wrong. Research has shown that, in some cases, these people are unhappy at home or at work. They are very depressed and so their backs hurt more than if they were happy. They don't need pain-killers, but they do need help sorting out their emotional problems.

More and more doctors are using a technique called visualization to help their patients feel better, even when they are seriously ill. Visualization does not make the disease go away but it helps people to cope with it better.

Suppose a man had a heart attack because the arteries to his heart were blocked. He could imagine an army of his cells rushing to the arteries armed with brooms and brushes to sweep and push away the blockage. By doing this he will be able to think about recovering instead of worrying about another heart attack.

SWITCHING OFF

Even when you are asleep your brain is still working, looking after the rest of your body. But everything slows down. Your brain makes your heart beat less often, you take fewer breaths, your muscles relax and food moves more slowly through your intestines.

The electrical signals from your brain also change. As you doze off, a few deep, slow waves appear among the normally fast, shallow electrical signals coming from your brain. Gradually the slow waves take over as you sleep. Once you are fully asleep you start to dream. Even though it may feel longer, you only dream for a few minutes every ninety minutes or so. Your eyes move quickly from side to side beneath your lids and other parts of your body may twitch too. Your brain waves are also fast and jerky.

Everyone needs sleep. It's when cells are renewed and the body repairs itself. The brain needs rest too – not to make new cells but to replace molecules, such as proteins, that it needs to work.

Without sleep, the brain soon suffers. People who do not have enough sleep cannot concentrate properly the next day. We can usually cope with one or two sleepless nights. The brain makes up for it the next night by spending more time in slow wave, deep sleep. But more than a few nights without sleep and we are in trouble!

Some people need less sleep than others. Most adults need seven to eight hours to feel refreshed and children need even more. But some people can get by with as little as three or four hours a night. Former British Prime Minister, Margaret Thatcher, only needed four hours.

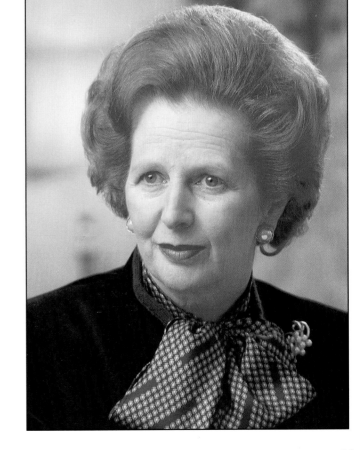

She was called the 'Iron Lady' because she was so tough. While everyone else was asleep in bed, the former British Prime Minister, Margaret Thatcher, was plotting her next political move.

There are lots of remedies for sleep problems (insomnia), including milky drinks, hot baths, reading a dull book and sleeping pills. It's best to try and avoid sleeping pills because people tend to depend on them too much. Many people with insomnia have other emotional problems which make it hard for them to sleep. They may be worried about their school work, their job, or their family, for example. Only when they sort these problems out will they be able to sleep normally.

A cup of coffee won't help her to sleep because the caffeine in it is a stimulant. But a hot milky drink without caffeine may help her to relax a bit.

TO SLEEP, PERCHANCE TO DREAM

For centuries, people have been trying to make sense of dreams. They read all sorts of things into them. But one new theory is that dreams are just a left-over from when we were in the womb. It is being suggested that the foetal brain stem sends the thinking parts of the brain – the grey matter – random signals before birth to get it used to the idea of working. But it doesn't stop doing it when we are born. It does it when we are asleep and our grey matter tries to make sense of the signals it is receiving by dipping into its memory banks. The result is gibberish!

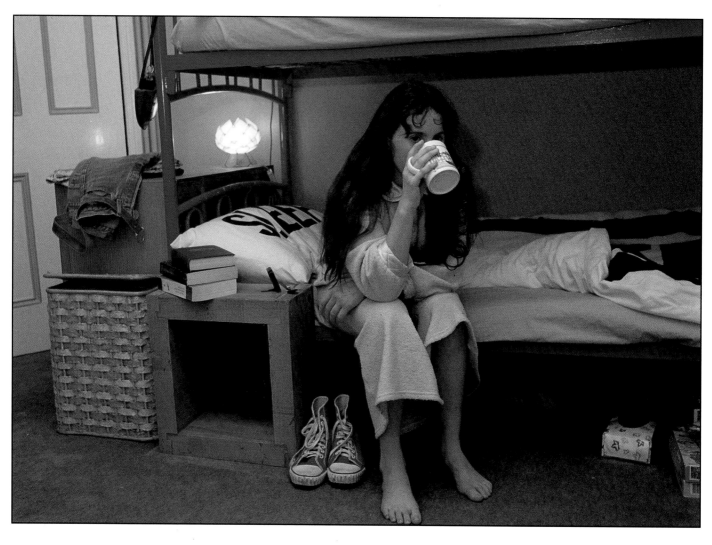

HEADACHES

Headaches are probably the most common ailment that humans get. But scientists know remarkably little about what causes them. Some people get more headaches than others. As many as one in five people suffer from a particular type of headache, called migraine. Until recently, scientists and doctors thought that only adults suffered from migraines. However, recent research has shown that children get them too.

Some headaches are blamed on tension in the muscles of the neck and head. Some follow hours watching television or reading a book. This may be due to focusing the eyes on one spot for too long. Some people get headaches when they are very hungry. Most adults have had a hangover headache at some time following too much alcohol. Whatever the cause, the result is the same – a throbbing pain in the head.

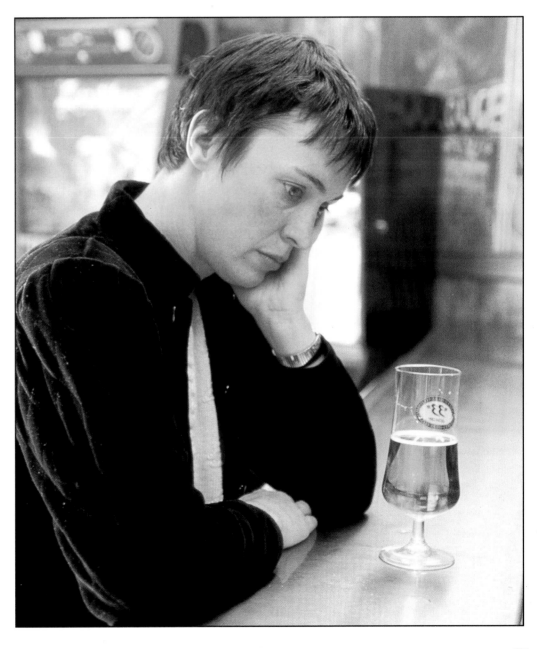

Is it worth the hangover? Alcohol has more effect on women, probably because they are smaller and have more fat and less water in their bodies than men.

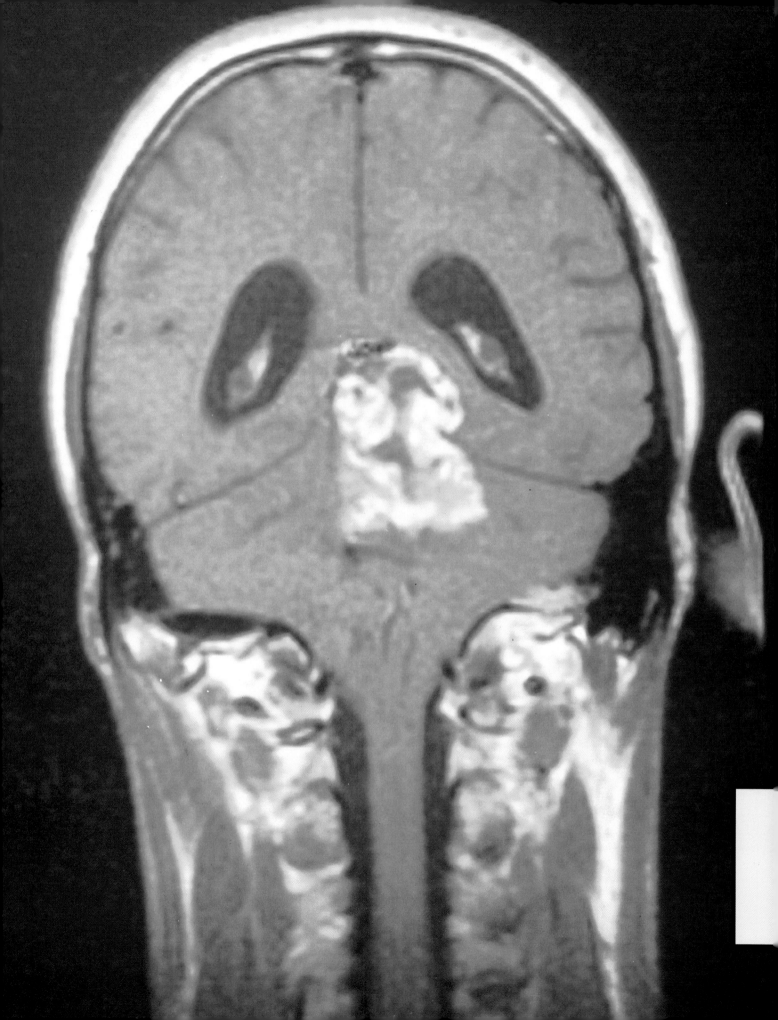

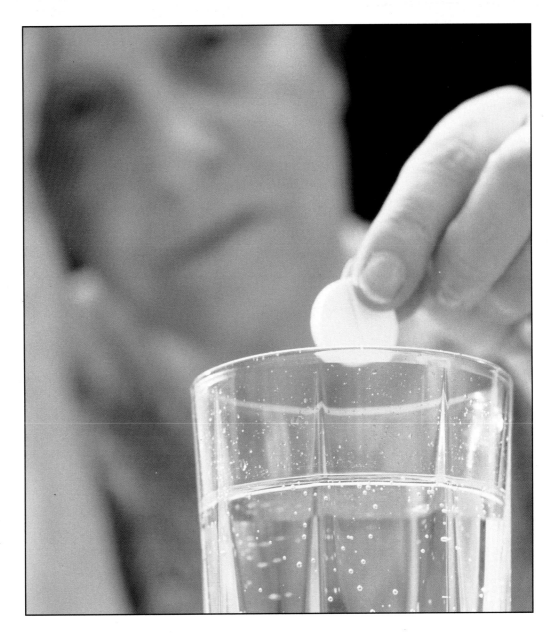

RIGHT Children under twelve should take paracetamol, not aspirin for a headache. In older people, paracetamol causes fewer stomach problems than aspirin.

OPPOSITE An X-ray of a man's brain, showing a tumour. This brain tumour (white part, centre) will be hard to remove surgically. But, luckily, doctors can often use powerful light rays to destroy brain tumours.

Most headaches can be cured with painkillers such as paracetamol or aspirin, but a migraine may need strong drugs. A migraine is thought to result from changes in the blood vessels and nerves of the brain. Sufferers may feel as though they have a tight band around their heads. Or the pain may be only on one side, above one eye. Often they are sick or they may see strange patterns. In fact, some migrane sufferers report hearing odd noises. However, this is extremely rare.

Strong painkillers can help but some people need other drugs to prevent attacks. If all else fails, many migraine sufferers find that if they can go to sleep in a darkened room they feel much better when they wake up.

All sorts of things can trigger a migraine, including certain foods like chocolate, red wine or cheese. So it's best to avoid these if they seem to make you worse.

BRAIN TUMOURS

Some people who have a lot of headaches worry that there might be something more serious wrong with them, such as a brain tumour. Fortunately, these are very rare. But anyone who is worried should be sure to see a doctor.

MENINGITIS

Meningitis is an infection of the delicate membranes which surround the brain. It can be caused by bacteria or viruses. It is most common in children and it is important to seek medical help as quickly as possible. An infected child usually has a high temperature, is drowsy and may be sick. Some have stiff necks.

Hospital tests can show what has caused the infection. If it is bacteria, antibiotics will cure it. Viral meningitis is more difficult to treat as anti-viral drugs are not very effective.

If meningitis is not treated it can lead to severe dehydration throughout the body which can be fatal. Anyone with the infection will be given

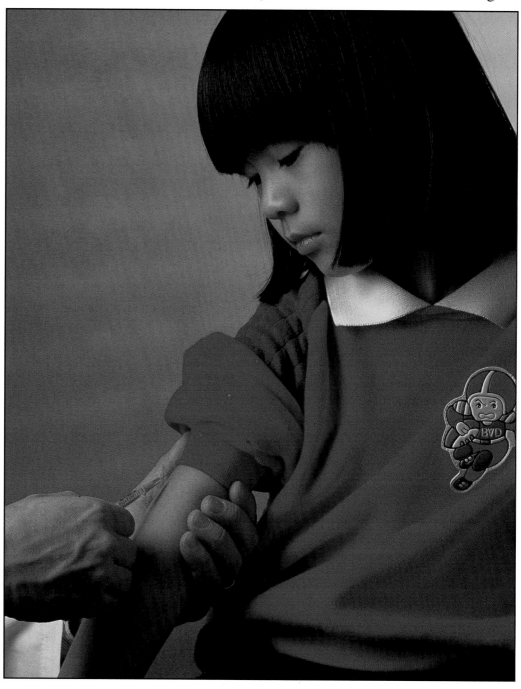

A new vaccine brought into use in 1992 is helping protect children against meningitis, but protection is not yet available against all the possible causes. Scientists are working on new vaccines.

lots of fluids into a vein in their arm to prevent dehydration.

Meningitis is infectious. If a child gets it, other children in his or her class may need to be given preventative treatment to stop them getting it too. This may mean them taking an antibiotic for a few days, or they may be vaccinated. Meningitis may be due to several different bacteria and viruses and the treatment given depends on the cause.

Most babies are immunized routinely against one of the bacteria that can cause meningitis. They have the vaccine at the same time as other routine childhood vaccines such as measles, mumps, German measles and whooping cough.

LUMBAR PUNCTURES

If a doctor thinks a child might have meningitis he or she will perform a lumbar puncture. This means taking a small sample of fluid from around the spinal cord. This fluid is called cerebrospinal fluid. It bathes the brain and spinal cord and helps to supply them with nutrients. It can become infected in meningitis. So doctors need to take a sample to look for bacteria or viruses. They can then give the most effective drugs for the kind of bacteria or viruses in question.

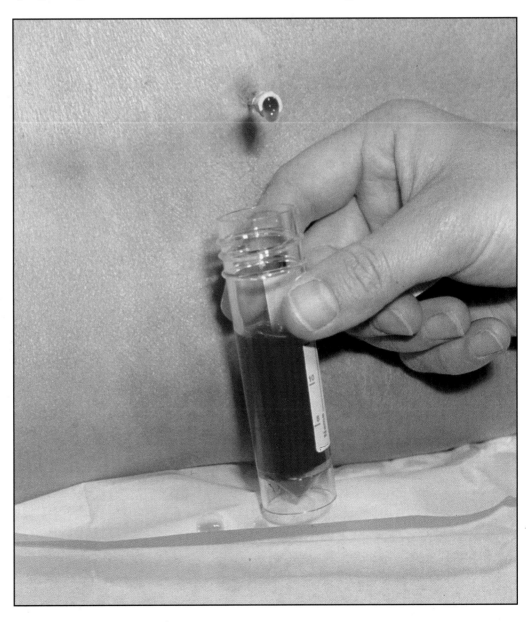

Fluid taken from this lumbar puncture has blood in it. This shows that part of the person's brain is bleeding.

EPILEPSY

Julius Caesar, Napoleon, Alfred Nobel and Byron are just a few of the 'greats' from history who had epilepsy. It didn't stop any of them getting to the top. Yet, people with epilepsy are sometimes treated as though they have an infectious disease. Other people are frightened of catching it. They are afraid they'll fall to the ground, foaming at the mouth. But most people with epilepsy lead totally normal lives. Thanks to modern drugs, many do not have epileptic fits from one year to the next.

Epilepsy affects about one in 200 people, one-third of them children. It can occur as a result of brain damage before, during or soon after birth. Sometimes it runs in families and is passed on from parent to child. If it occurs later, it is more likely to be a result of infection. Epilepsy can also start in old age, usually following a stroke.

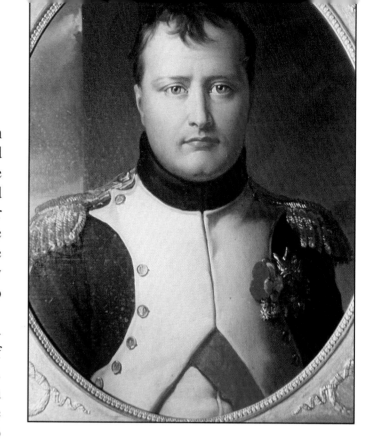

ABOVE Epilepsy didn't stop Napoleon.

RIGHT Doctors learn how to interpret electrical recordings of brain activity. This recording revealed epilepsy. Can you spot the abnormal spikes on rows 6, 13, 14 and 15?

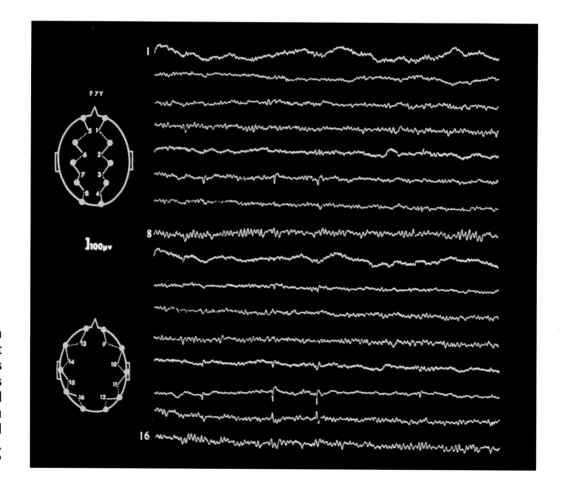

When doctors test the electrical signals from brain cells of people with epilepsy they find that they are abnormal. It seems that the cells become over-excited.

If only a small area of the brain is affected, spasms only occur in the part of the body controlled by it. If more of the brain is involved, spasms may affect more of the body and the person may become unconscious.

There are several drugs that are prescribed by doctors to control epilepsy and prevent attacks. In most cases they are very effective. Occasionally however, the drugs are not enough and an operation may be needed. Recently doctors have realized that people can learn how to control, prevent or delay their fits when they feel them coming on. They can also avoid things that can bring on an attack, like flashing lights.

WHAT TO DO IF SOMEONE HAS A FIT

Don't panic or run away. If possible turn the person on to their stomach with their head on one side so they can breath properly (see below). Move furniture out of harm's way. Don't try to hold the person down or put anything in their mouth. Send someone to get help. Or, if you are on your own, wait for the fit to stop.

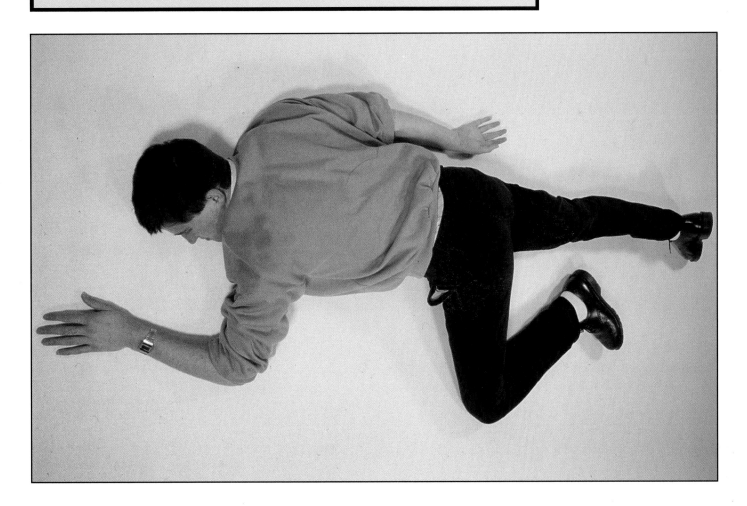

HEAD INJURIES

If you fall over and bang your head be sure to tell whoever is looking after you. You may think your head is pretty hard but your brain is delicate. Like any other part of your body, it may bleed if it is bumped or cut.

If you cut your hand, put some antiseptic cream on it and perhaps a plaster. If the cut is deep you may need some stitches. But if you cut your brain you won't know that it is bleeding. If it bleeds a lot there may be serious damage. If you get a headache after you bang your head or you are sick, feel ill or have a temperature you should see a doctor straight away. He or she will probably advise you to have an X-ray or a brain scan to check there's no serious damage. If there is some bleeding inside your head it is sometimes necessary to have an operation to stop the bleeding and patch up any damage that has been done.

Always protect your head when you are riding a bicycle or doing something else where you could damage it, such as horse riding or rock climbing. Get yourself a helmet that fits you properly and look for a symbol confirming that it has passed the government's safety checks.

If you take part in sports such as boxing, don't be tempted to fight, even for a few minutes, without head protection. Each time your head is punched your brain moves from side to side within the skull and this can cause permanent damage. Many professional boxers have been physically or mentally damaged because they have taken too many blows to the head.

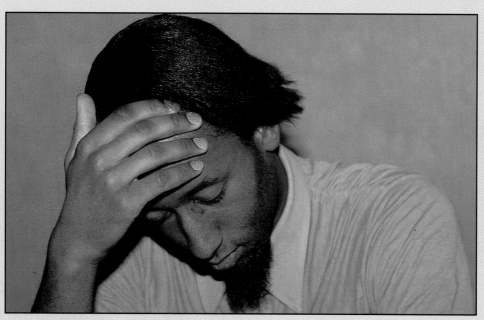

FAINTING

Have you ever fainted? It's a bit of a shock when you suddenly find yourself on the floor! People faint when there isn't enough blood getting to their brains. This can happen if they get up too suddenly or their blood pressure is low for some other reason. If you feel faint, either sit down with your head between your knees or lie down with your feet up on a box or low chair.

OPPOSITE This climber's safety helmet could mean the difference between a nasty concussion and permanent brain damage if he falls. Don't take unnecessary risks, it's not worth it.

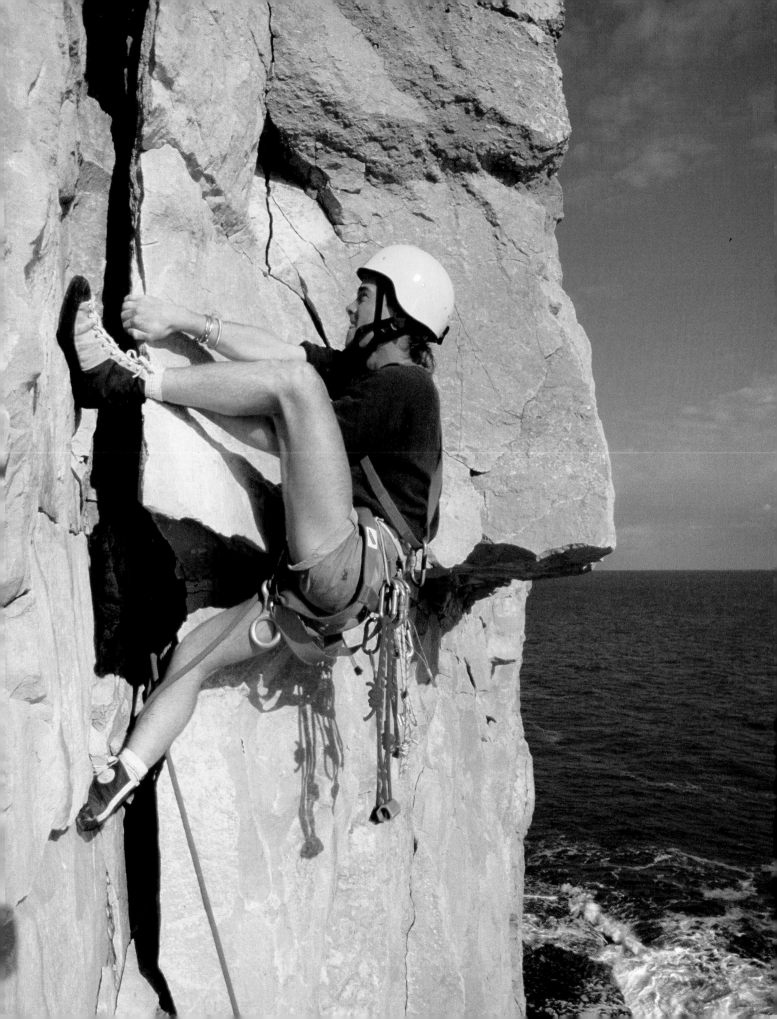

ANXIETY AND DEPRESSION

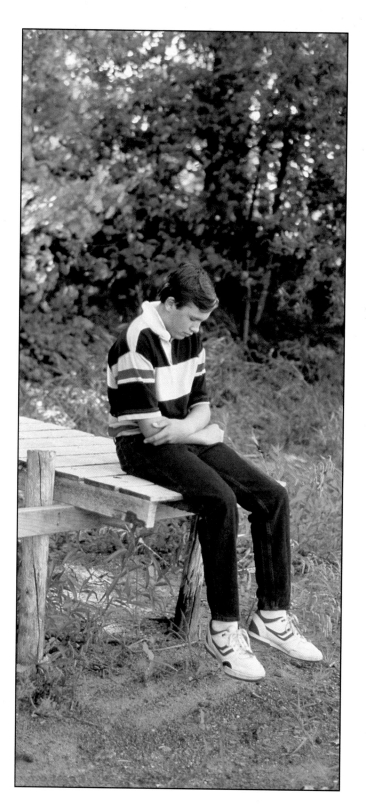

How often does someone tell you that you get on their nerves? Perhaps you have a picture of whizzing down wires in their body, like riding down the bannisters of a staircase! What they really mean when they say this is that you are making them cross, irritable and anxious.

We all know what it's like to get anxious. You probably get jittery before you take an exam or before going on stage in the school play. But imagine what it would be like to be worried every minute of the day.

Most people who suffer from anxiety have a problem at work or at home. They may be worried that they are going to lose their job or they may not get on with their boss. They may be having rows with their husband or wife or one of their children may be in trouble at school.

This builds up to make them feel anxious. They can't concentrate so they fall behind at work. They may forget to do things, or they may lie awake at night worrying. All this makes the anxiety worse.

Anxiety is sometimes mixed up with depression because the symptoms are similar. Depressed people may also get anxious, but they tend to be more unhappy and unable to cope with life. Sometimes women get depressed after having a baby – this is called having the 'baby blues'.

It's natural to feel fed up from time to time. But it is not normal for someone to feel depressed all the time, often for no reason.

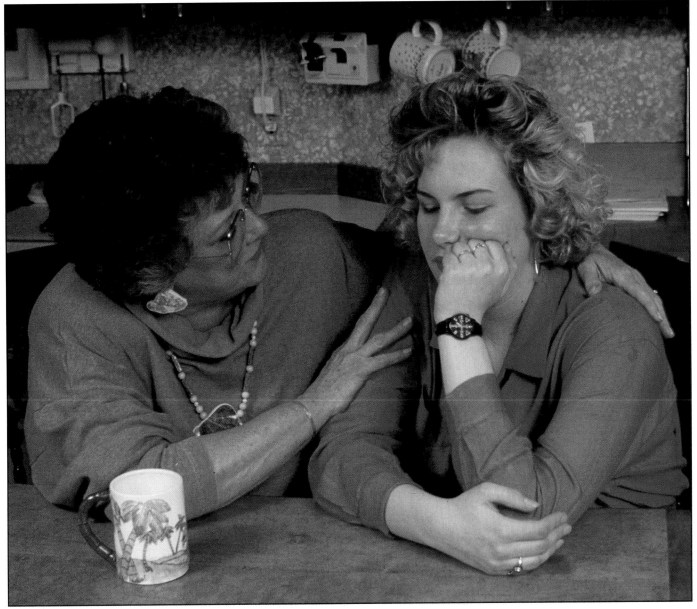

Don't bottle up your troubles. Tell someone else what's on your mind.

The best treatment is to sort out the problems that are causing the anxiety or depression. This may mean talking the problems over with your family and friends or with a professional counsellor who is trained to help.

People with depression are more likely to need drugs to help them. These can be taken for a few weeks or months and they are usually very effective. In general, people who suffer from anxiety are now advised to avoid drugs. This is because the drugs most commonly used to treat anxiety can be extremely addictive.

COMING OFF TRANQUILLIZERS

About ten years ago, doctors realized that tranquillizer drugs commonly used to treat anxiety were addictive. People felt agitated and ill, and some even had hallucinations when they tried to stop taking them. People who want to stop taking drugs for anxiety should talk to their doctors so the dose can be reduced slowly. This way, they are less likely to get withdrawal symptoms.

A CRY FOR HELP

Every year a small number of teenagers commit suicide. Others try to kill themselves but are saved. How do they get to the point where death seems to be the only way out? When was the last time you felt really unhappy? What made you feel so miserable? Was it something at school or at home? Was someone nasty to you?

BELOW Don't make life miserable for someone in your class. Think how you'd feel if people were nasty to you.

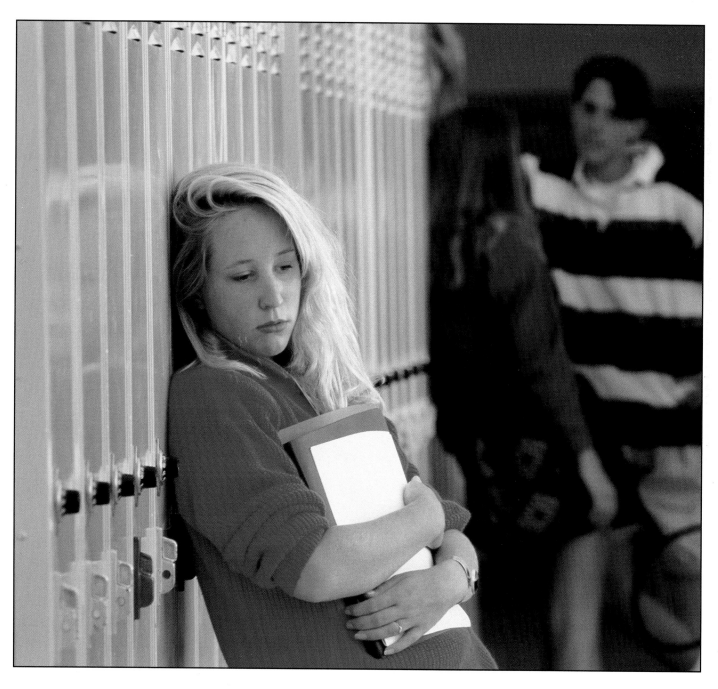

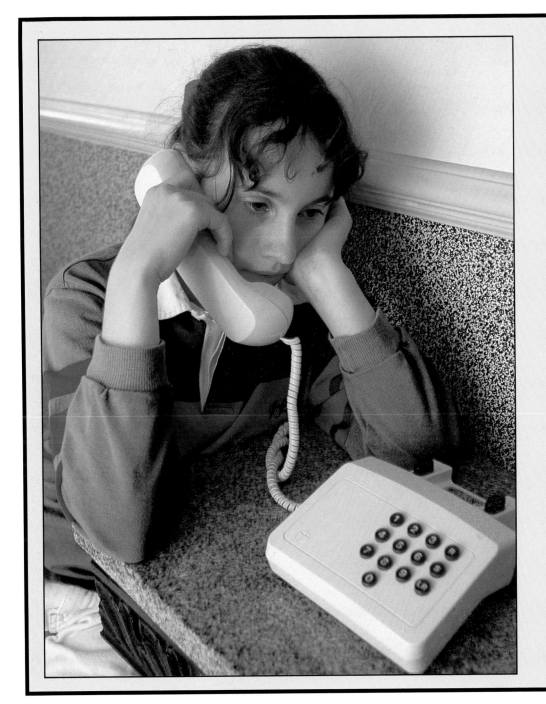

HELPLINES

If you would rather talk about your problems with someone who does not know you, you can contact a group like the Samaritans. They are in the phone book. There are other groups that have been set up just to help children. Again, look in your phone book. They may be listed at the front with the emergency services. Or you can ask the operator to help you.

Perhaps there are posters with helpful numbers on your school noticeboard. If you phone one of these groups they will help you. They won't tell anyone about your call unless you say that they can.

There are lots of things you can do to help when you are upset. It's best not to bottle things up. If you let things out, you'll always feel a lot better. You can go home and have a good cry. There's nothing wrong with that.

You can talk to someone about your problems. That could be your mother or father, brother or sister or a friend. They may not be able to make it better. But you'll find that talking helps. You may be able to work out an answer to your problem.

If you are miserable because you are being bullied – or you know someone who is being bullied – you should tell an adult, either your parents or a teacher. It's not telling tales. And you'll be surprised how grateful your friends will be. A bully doesn't just pick on one person. He or she usually does it again and again. Others in your class know that they could be next to suffer. So they'll be glad if the bully is found out and his or her cruelty stopped.

SAY NO!

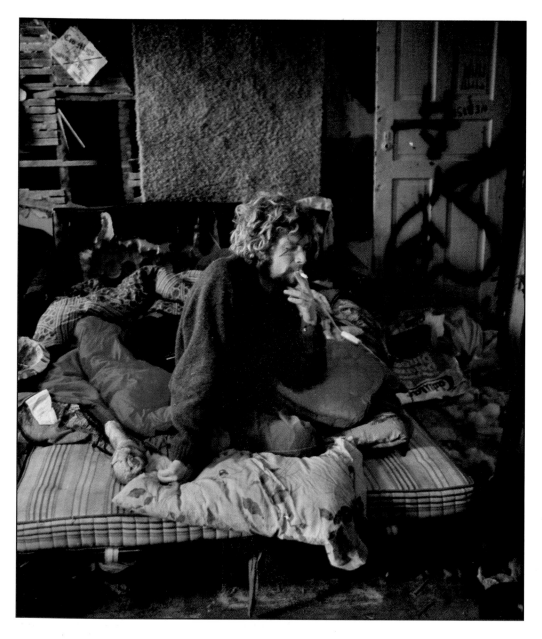

Don't end up like this. Don't kid yourself that you can stop when you want to – you will get hooked. Say no to all drugs.

Alcohol, heroin, glue, cocaine and LSD are just a few of the drugs that affect the brain and can cause lasting damage. People take drugs like these for lots of reasons – to make them feel better, to shut out things they don't want to think about or simply because their friends do.

Some of these drugs, like alcohol, glue and heroin, make people feel relaxed. Their speech becomes slurred and they can't focus their eyes. ... can't concentrate and they feel sleepy. Other drugs, such as cocaine and amphetamines, make people feel excited. They need less sleep and they want to be very active.

Some amphetamines and drugs like LSD and 'magic mushrooms' make people hallucinate. They may feel excited or frightened, depending on what their hallucinations are like. Cannabis – the most widely misused illegal drug – also has mixed effects. Sometimes it makes people relaxed and drowsy and, at other times, excited and talkative.

Drinking too much alcohol or taking any of these drugs doesn't just damage the brain. It affects the way you behave. Someone who is drunk or high on drugs may do things that he or she wouldn't dream of doing normally. Suddenly, they may become violent, or abusive. Or they may think they can fly off a roof top or run in front of a car without getting killed. If they are driving they may take risks that could kill themselves and other people. You cannot reason with someone who is drunk or taking drugs. They do not understand or think logically.

Those who take addictive drugs become slaves to their habits. Their brain cells cannot do without the drugs and if they don't take them they become mentally and physically ill. Getting their drugs comes first. Their jobs, their families, their friends and their homes don't matter any more.

HOW TO SAY NO

Have you ever been offered drugs? What did you say? Sometimes it's hard to say no. Your friends may be taking drugs and you feel stupid if you are left out. But they are the stupid ones. They are making themselves ill and risking other people's lives too. In a few years time you'll be pitying them, not envying them. So, say no!

BELOW Acid house parties and 'raves' are easy targets for drug pushers. Just enjoy the music instead.

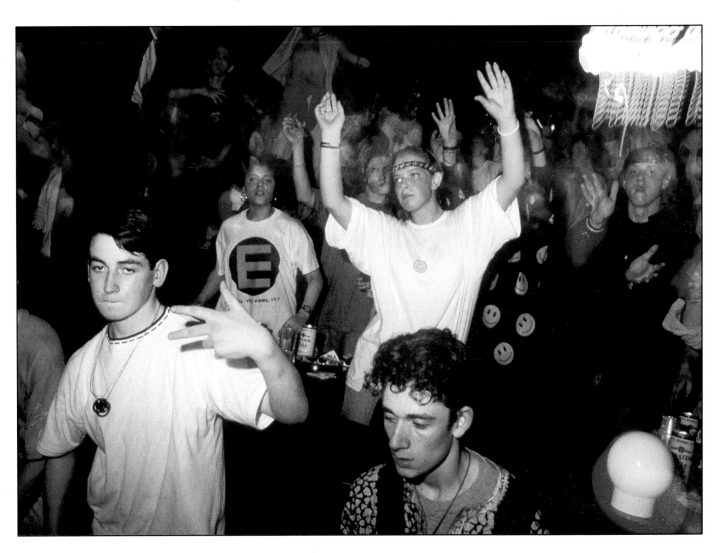

MAD OR BAD?

A fourteen-year-old boy throws acid in the face of an elderly widow and steals £4 from her purse. A fifteen-year-old girl smothers her newborn baby and puts the body in the dustbin.

How can they do such terrible things? Are they mad and in need of our help? Or are they bad and should they be locked up?

Let's find out some more about them. Kevin, the fourteen-year-old boy, has lived most of his life in children's homes. He was put in care at the age of four because his parents beat him. Since then, two sets of foster parents have said they do not want him because he is too difficult. He has been using drugs since he was ten.

Can we help Kevin or is it too late? Should we try and find a family who will take him in? Or should we lock him up and teach him a lesson?

Suppose Kevin came from a loving family who had always given him everything he wanted. But he still threw acid in the old lady's face. Should we treat him differently from the Kevin who had a miserable childhood?

BELOW Special schemes, such as this one, have been very successful in helping people to lead better lives.

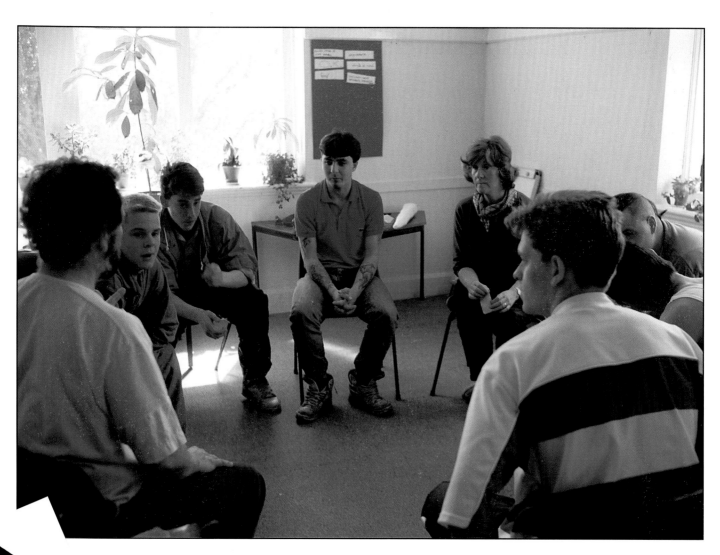

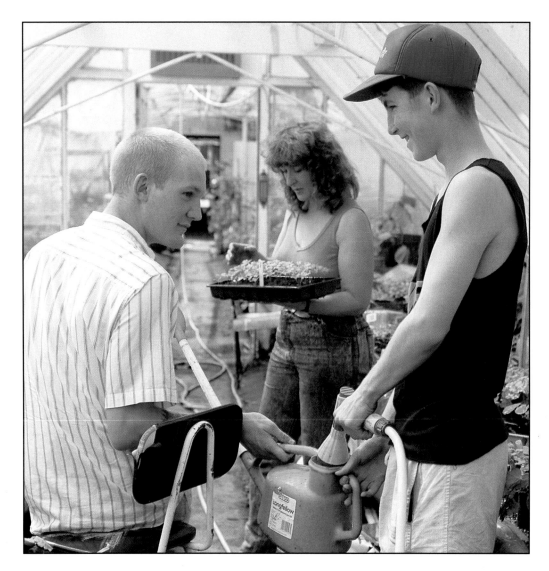

Let's hear about Cathy, the fifteen-year-old who killed her baby. She came from a hard-working family. There wasn't much money for holidays but Cathy always had the best her parents could give her. When they found out she was pregnant they were very upset. But they said they would look after the baby while she finished school and got her exams.

Can we forgive Cathy for what she did? Her parents were going to help her. Was she mad when she killed her baby, or wicked?

Suppose Cathy had been less fortunate. She had run away from home and lived rough in a big city. She didn't know anyone who could help her. Should we forgive her now?

There are many similar shocking stories about teenagers like Kevin and Cathy in the newspapers.

How would you help them and stop others from doing such terrible things?

DR JEKYLL OR MR HYDE?

In Robert Louis Stevenson's famous book, *The Strange Case of Dr Jekyll and Mr Hyde*, Dr Jekyll was a kind caring doctor. But when he swallowed a drug he was experimenting with, he turned into Mr Hyde – a vicious murderer. In real life, people don't have this sort of split personality. But some do experience big changes in mood – sometimes happy and excited, sometimes miserable and depressed. They may need medical help.

MENTAL ILLNESS

In the nineteenth century and for most of the twentieth century, people with serious mental illnesses were looked after in large mental hospitals, called asylums. Some were put there by relatives for quite minor illnesses because they were too embarrassed to have them at home. Others were too ill to cope at home and there were few drugs to treat their illnesses.

Once someone was in an asylum it was very difficult to get out. Some were too frightened to come out even when they were better. They had forgotten how to look after themselves.

Towards the end of the 1960s, many governments decided that mentally ill people should be cared for at home or in smaller centres in more friendly, personal environments.

The idea was to provide 'sheltered' homes. People with mental illnesses and disabilities would live in small groups in houses where there were people who could help them. They would be encouraged to shop, cook and care for themselves and, where possible, to get jobs. Those who couldn't work would go to day centres where they would be given simple tasks and looked after by a team of helpers.

Unfortunately, there are rarely enough sheltered homes. Some people cannot cope even in this type of care. Or they go home only to find their families cannot cope with them. They forget to take their drugs and their illnesses get worse. They go off on their own and many live rough in big cities with no one to look after them.

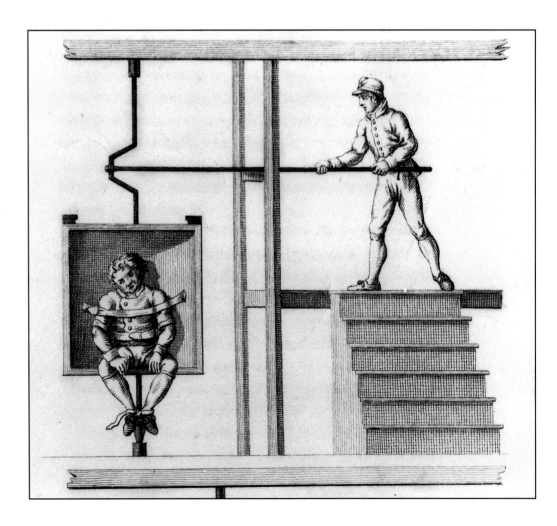

It's hard to believe that in the nineteenth century, mentally ill patients were sometimes whirled around in chairs or beds to and shake some nse into them!

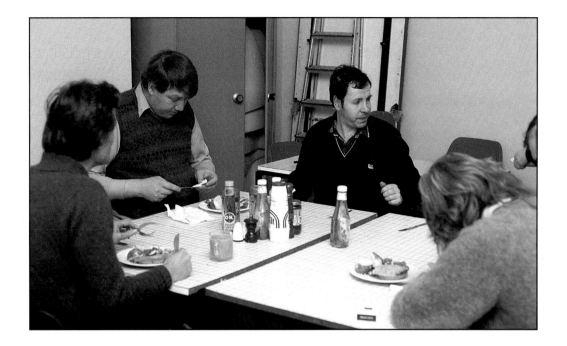

LEFT Today, some mentally ill people go to day centres where they are given food and looked after.

HOMELESS PEOPLE

Most people who live rough in big cities would prefer to have a home of their own. A few like to live this way. Each night they go to sleep in boxes or sleeping bags in shop doorways, under bridges, in parks – anywhere with shelter from the wind and rain.

Whose fault is it that they have nowhere to go?

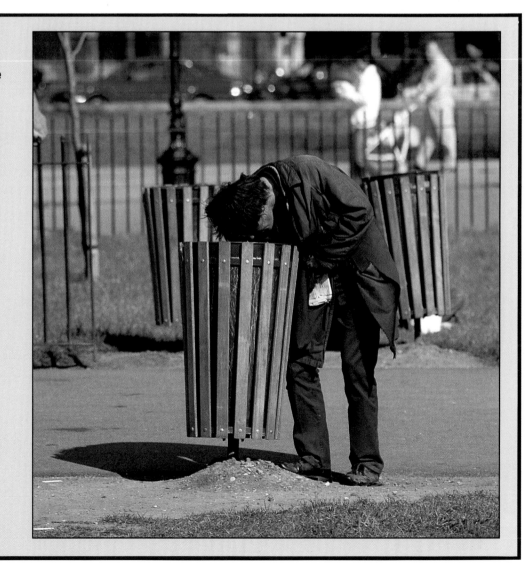

GLOSSARY

cerebellum the area of the brain that deals with movement and balance.

chromosomes thread-like structures found in all body cells. They carry genes which determine what a person is like.

conception when an egg is fertilized by a sperm.

cortex outer layer of the brain.

dehydration huge loss of water from the body which can lead to coma and death.

embryo unborn child in the womb, from two to eight weeks after conception. After eight weeks and until birth it is called a foetus.

evolution development of species over millions of years; some species have become more advanced than others.

genes tiny parts of chromosomes that determine what a person is like.

grey matter brain cells needed for thinking.

membrane thin layer of tissue which acts as a wall in the body and may protect delicate organs underneath.

myelin white coating which covers nerves that carry messages long distances. It makes messages move more quickly.

personality a person's characteristics, such as whether they laugh a lot, are nasty or kind. Everyone's personality is different.

spasm an uncontrolled movement in part of the body.

species group of organisms, such as humans or dogs which look like each other and can reproduce by mating with others of the same species.

white matter nerve fibres in the brain that look white because they are covered in myelin. They carry messages between cells.

BOOKS TO READ

Moods and Feelings by John Coleman
(Wayland, 1990)
Your Brain and Nervous System by D.
Baldwin (Wayland, 1986)
The Use of Drugs by Brian Ward
(Macdonald, 1986)
Drugs and Medicine by Jenny Bryan
(Wayland, 1992)

The Body and How it Works by Steve Parker
(Dorling Kindersley, 1987)
Be Positive! by Miriam Moss (Wayland, 1992)
Twentieth Century Medicine by Jenny Bryan
(Wayland, 1988)
The Human Body by Ruth and Bertel Bruun
(Kingfisher Books, 1987)

ACKNOWLEDGEMENTS

Sally & Richard Greenhill 42, 43, 45 (top); National Medical Slide Bank 10, 33; Rex Features Ltd 13, 17 (Craig Easton), 23, 24 (Rick Colls), 26 (Rick Colls), 32, 39 (Rick Colls); Science Photo Library 7 (M. Abbey), 8 (Petit Format/Nestle), 12 (M. Abbey), 14 (Keane/BSIP), 19 (Hank Morgan), 21 (Carlos Goldin), 27 (BSIP Zarand), 28 (Simon Fraser/Neuroradiology Department/Newcastle General Hospital), 31 (Biophoto Associates), 33, 44 (National Library of Medicine); Skjold 5, 15 (bottom), 16, 22, 36, 37; Tony Stone Worldwide 25 (Ed Pritchard), 30 (Tom Raymond), 35 (Oli Tennent), 38 (David Ximeno Tejada); Topham 4, 40, 41; Zefa cover/title page, 9, 15 (top), 18, 45.
Artwork: Malcolm S. Walker.

INDEX